ANTI-INFLAMMATORY
COOKBOOK FOR BEGINNERS

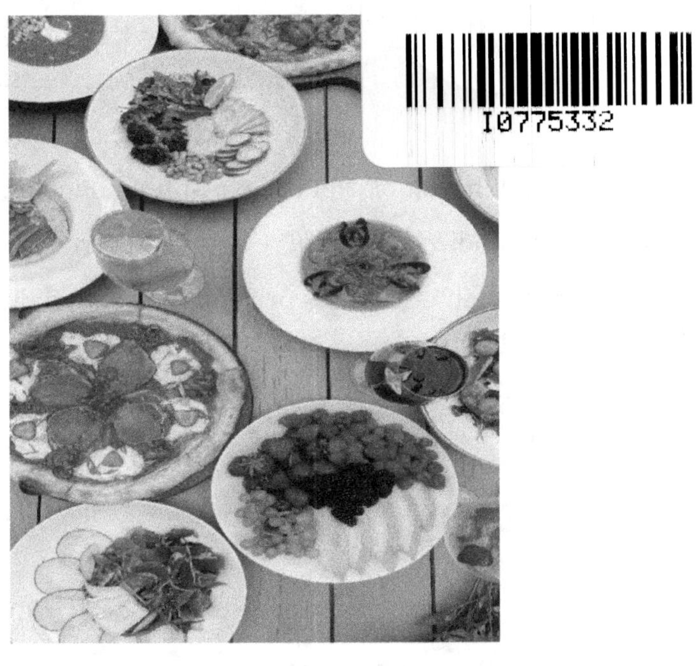

Discover Wellness - Tasty Recipes for

Healthy Living

Angela W. Ashley

Table of content

INTRODUCTION

In the hectic center of the city, where the fast-paced lifestyle frequently has a detrimental impact on our wellbeing, a journey to vibrant health and energy via the magic of anti-inflammatory cooking is waiting to be discovered. Hello and welcome to Anti-Inflammatory Cuisine, where each recipe serves as a step toward reducing inflammation and embracing a healthy lifestyle.

Inflammation has become an unwelcome companion for many people in the midst of modern life's hustle and bustle. Stress, processed foods, and sedentary lives have all contributed to our misery, leaving us seeking for relief. This cookbook was prepared during the search for a comprehensive solution; it is intended to assist both expert cooks and anyone desiring to begin a tasty route to an inflammation-free life.

As you turn the pages, you'll discover the power of components chosen expressly for their ability to alleviate inflammation. Consider a world in which each bite is a harmonious combination of nutrients and flavors that nourish your body from the inside out. Consider a bright food table that will not only excite your mouth but also feed your cells, leaving you feeling revitalized and energized.

We begin our journey by looking deeply into the science of inflammation and its impact on our health. From there, we make our way into the kitchen's heart, where sophistication and simplicity meet. The "Anti-inflammatory Cookbook for Beginners" promotes the notion that healthy cooking does not have to be complicated. Using easy recipes and widely available ingredients, even the most inexperienced cook may create wonderful anti-inflammatory foods.

The cookbook is more than just a collection of recipes; it is a guide to redefining your relationship with food. Every meal tells a story, a testament to the healing properties of healthy foods. Every ingredient, from the delicate aroma of fresh herbs to the earthy notes of turmeric, has been carefully chosen for its ability to reduce inflammation and promote wellbeing.

Introducing Sarah, a busy professional who found the life-changing effects of anti-inflammatory cooking after years of suffering from acute tiredness. Her story, which is interwoven throughout the book, demonstrates the transformational impact of eating anti-inflammatory foods. As she makes her way through the recipes, Sarah develops a newfound pleasure for cooking, soothing herself in the knowledge that her meals are now an occasion for self-care as well as food.

The "Anti-inflammatory Cookbook for Beginners" places as much emphasis on eating behaviors as it does on substance. The cookbook introduces readers to mindful eating strategies, encouraging them to savor every bite, notice the flavors and textures, and live in the now. This allows people to create a stronger contact with their bodies and promotes harmony in their lives.

So, regardless of your level of culinary experience or desire to embrace a healthy lifestyle, the cookbook encourages you to enter a world where food becomes medicine and every meal is an opportunity to nurture your body and spirit. Allow the flavors to dance on your tongue and the aroma of anti-inflammatory spices to fill your kitchen. Greetings from the beginning of a wonderful journey toward a life of health and vitality.

CHAPTER 1:

UNDERSTANDING ANTI-INFLAMMATORY

Anti-inflammatory in a lay-man term.

Anti-inflammatory actions or substances aid in the reduction of inflammation in the body. Inflammation is the body's normal response to injury or infection, but it can lead to a variety of health problems when it becomes chronic. Anti-inflammatory strategies, such as certain diets or lifestyle choices, help to alleviate this chronic inflammation. Consider it a calming balm for your skin; these acts help to alleviate redness, swelling, and discomfort. Choosing an anti-inflammatory diet entails consuming foods high in antioxidants, omega-3 fatty acids, and colorful fruits and vegetables. By adopting this strategy, you are doing more than just eating; you are making decisions that will help your body feel its best and sustain long-term health.

How does inflammatory affect patient's life?

- Inflammation often causes pain and discomfort in numerous places of the body. Discomfort, whether from joint pain, muscle pains, or headaches, can have a substantial impact on a patient's everyday life, reducing movement and general well-being.

- The body's ongoing fight against inflammation can lead to chronic weariness. Even after adequate rest, patients may have a lack of vitality, which can interfere with job, social activities, and personal relationships.

- Inflammation can disturb sleep patterns, making it harder to fall or stay asleep. Poor sleep quality exacerbates exhaustion and can lead to an inflammatory cycle, creating a difficult circle for patients.

- Mood disorders such as anxiety and depression have been linked to inflammatory diseases. Inflammation's physical toll, paired with its effect on neurotransmitters, can add to emotional difficulties, impacting a patient's mental health and resilience.

- Inflammation of the gastrointestinal tract can cause digestive problems such abdominal pain, bloating, and irregular bowel movements. Patients may experience not only physical discomfort but also emotional suffering as a result of these symptoms.

- Some inflammatory disorders, especially those that impact the brain, might cause cognitive deficits. Memory, focus, and overall cognitive function issues may influence a patient's ability to accomplish tasks that require mental acuity.

- Chronic inflammation can weaken the immune system, leaving the body vulnerable to infections and disorders. This increased susceptibility to external dangers might result in more frequent illnesses, negatively impacting a patient's overall health and lifestyle.

- Chronic inflammation can cause joint stiffness and decreased flexibility in muscles and tissues. This limitation in mobility impacts not just physical activity but also one's capacity to accomplish normal duties, lowering one's overall quality of life.

What is an anti-inflammatory cookbook?

Anti-inflammatory cookbook for beginners is a culinary guide aimed to ease and enrich one's journey toward a healthier living. This cookbook exposes novice cooks to a palate of tasty, easy-to-make foods that highlight anti-inflammatory ingredients, with the goal of lowering inflammation in the body. Each cuisine, from vivid veggies to nutrient-rich proteins and hearty fats, is a step toward better health. Beyond only great recipes, the cookbook also functions as an instructional tool, arming newcomers with knowledge about the science of inflammation. It elevates cooking from a chore to a pleasurable, health-conscious experience, creating the groundwork for long-term vigor and balanced nutrition.

Can good dieting improve the well-being of an inflammatory patient?

- Adopting an anti-inflammatory diet high in fruits, vegetables, leafy greens, and berries can supply critical vitamins, minerals, and antioxidants that fight inflammation at the cellular level.

- Lean proteins supply vital amino acids while avoiding saturated fats, which may contribute to inflammation. Choosing lean protein sources such as poultry, fish, tofu, and beans can aid with inflammation management.

- Choosing healthy grains over processed carbohydrates helps to reduce inflammation. Whole grains contain fiber and minerals that promote intestinal health and inflammatory regulation.

- Consuming a varied range of phytonutrients and antioxidants, which play an important role in lowering inflammation and promoting general health, is ensured by eating a variety of colorful vegetables.

- Incorporating omega-3 fatty acid sources into the diet can have powerful anti-inflammatory effects since omega-3s assist in regulating the body's inflammatory response and enhance overall cardiovascular health.

- Incorporating sources of healthy fats, such as olive oil, avocados, and almonds, into your diet will help you maintain an anti-inflammatory diet. These fats have been related to reduce inflammatory levels in the body.

- Patients can improve their metabolic health and reduce their inflammatory indicators by limiting their intake of sugary meals and beverages.

Frequently asked questions by anti-inflammatory patients.

- **What exactly is inflammation, and why does it happen in the body?** It is the body's natural response to damage or infection which involves immune cells, blood vessels, and chemical mediators. Its goal is to remove the source of cell harm, clear away damaged cells, and begin tissue restoration.

- **What are some of the most common signs of chronic inflammation?** Chronic inflammation can express itself in a variety of ways, including chronic pain, swelling, exhaustion, and frequent illness. It may also play a role in the development of ailments such as arthritis, cardiovascular disease, and autoimmune disorders.

- **How do I tell the difference between acute and chronic inflammation?** Acute inflammation is a short-term reaction to injury or illness that causes redness, swelling, and pain. Chronic inflammation, on the other hand, lasts longer and does not always display obvious signs, making it critical to check for underlying health concerns.

- **How can diet affect inflammation?** Diet has a significant impact on either generating or decreasing inflammation. An anti-inflammatory diet high in fruits, vegetables, omega-3 fatty acids, and whole grains can help reduce inflammation, but diets high in processed foods and sugars can aggravate it.

- **Are there particular foods that can assist in reducing inflammation?** Certain foods, in fact, have anti-inflammatory effects. These include fatty fish, leafy green, berries, turmeric, and antioxidant-rich meals.

CHAPTER 2: BREAKFAST RECIPES

Quinoa Breakfast Porridge:

<u>Ingredients</u>: Quinoa, coconut milk, cinnamon, fresh berries, honey.

<u>Instructions</u>:

- Add a sprinkle of cinnamon to cooked quinoa in coconut milk.
- Add some fresh berries to the mixture.
- Drizzle honey over the top.

<u>Prep Time</u>: 20 minutes

<u>Nutritional Information</u>: Protein, fiber and antioxidants

Avocado Toast with Poached Egg:

<u>Ingredients</u>: Whole grain bread, avocado, poached egg, cherry tomatoes, salt, pepper.

<u>Instructions</u>:

- Make a toast and sprinkle avocado mash on it.
- Add sliced cherry tomatoes and a poached egg on top.
- Add pepper and salt for seasoning.

<u>Prep Time</u>: 10 minutes

<u>Nutritional Information</u>: Healthy fats, protein, and vitamins.

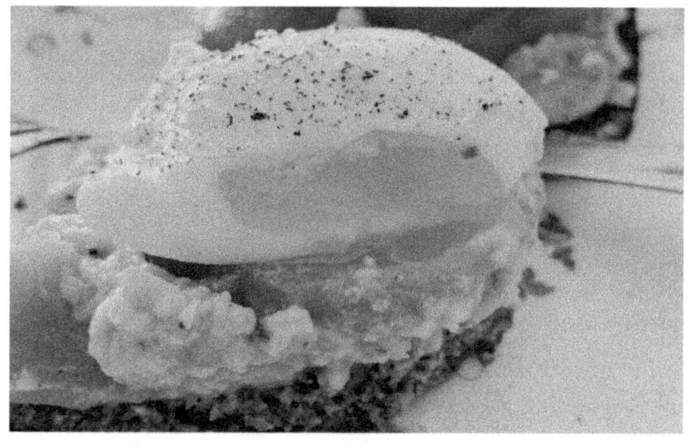

Chia Seed Pudding Parfait:

<u>Ingredients</u>: Chia seeds, almond milk, vanilla extract, Greek yogurt, mixed berries.

Instructions:

- Combine almond milk, vanilla essence, and chia seeds.
- Let it settle for the night.
- Add mixed berries and Greek yogurt to the layer.

Prep Time: 5 minutes (plus overnight soaking)

Nutritional Information: Protein, omega-3s and antioxidants

Oatmeal with Turmeric and Berries:

Ingredients: Rolled oats, turmeric, almond milk, mixed berries, honey.

Instructions:

- Boil oats in almond milk with turmeric.
- Add a drizzle of honey and a mixture of berries on top.

Prep Time: 15 minutes

Nutritional Information: Fiber, antioxidants, and anti-inflammatory properties.

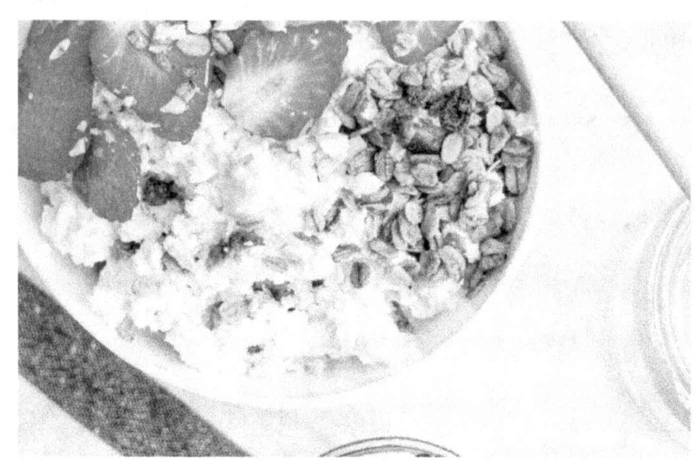

Mushroom and Spinach Breakfast Wrap:

<u>Ingredients</u>: Whole grain wrap, sautéed mushrooms, spinach, scrambled eggs.

<u>Instructions</u>:

- Prepare a grain wrap.
- Top the grain wrap with sautéed mushrooms, spinach, and scrambled eggs.
- Serve and enjoy.

<u>Prep Time</u>: 15 minutes

Nutritional Information: Protein, fiber, and vitamins.

Sweet Potato and Spinach Frittata:

Ingredients: Eggs, sweet potatoes, spinach, red bell pepper, feta cheese.

Instructions:

- Sauté the red bell pepper, spinach, and sweet potatoes.
- Cover the vegetables with whisked eggs
- Sprinkle feta over the top, and bake until set.

Prep Time: 25 minutes

Nutritional Information: Protein, vitamin A, and iron.

Cauliflower and Kale Breakfast Hash:

Ingredients: Cauliflower, kale, red onion, garlic, poached egg.

Instructions:

- Sauté the garlic, red onion, kale, and cauliflower.
- Add a poached egg on top.

<u>Prep Time</u>: 20 minutes

<u>Nutritional Information</u>: Low-carb, high fiber, and vitamins.

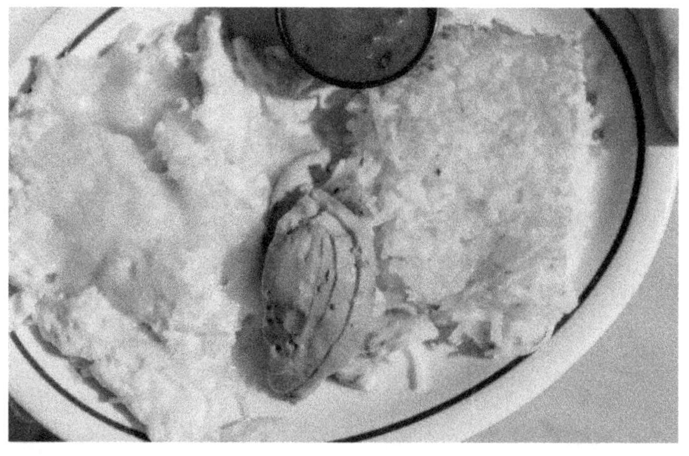

Green Tea Chia Pudding:

<u>Ingredients</u>: Green tea, chia seeds, almond milk, honey.

<u>Instructions</u>:

- Make a cup of green tea.
- Add almond milk and chia seeds.
- After letting it set, drizzle with honey.

<u>Prep Time</u>: 10 minutes (plus soaking time)

<u>Nutritional Information</u>: Antioxidants, omega-3s, and fiber.

Tomato and Basil Breakfast Quinoa:

<u>Ingredients</u>: Quinoa, cherry tomatoes, fresh basil, feta cheese.

<u>Instructions</u>:

- Prepare the quinoa.
- Combine it with fresh basil, feta cheese, and half of the cherry tomatoes.
- Serve and savor!

<u>Prep Time</u>: 15 minutes

<u>Nutritional Information</u>: Protein, vitamin C, and calcium.

Almond and Blueberry Protein Pancakes:

<u>Ingredients</u>: Almond flour, eggs, blueberries, almond milk.

<u>Instructions</u>:

- Combine almond flour, eggs, blueberries, and almond milk.
- Fry as pancakes.

<u>Prep Time</u>: 15 minutes

<u>Nutritional Information</u>: Protein, antioxidants, and healthy fats.

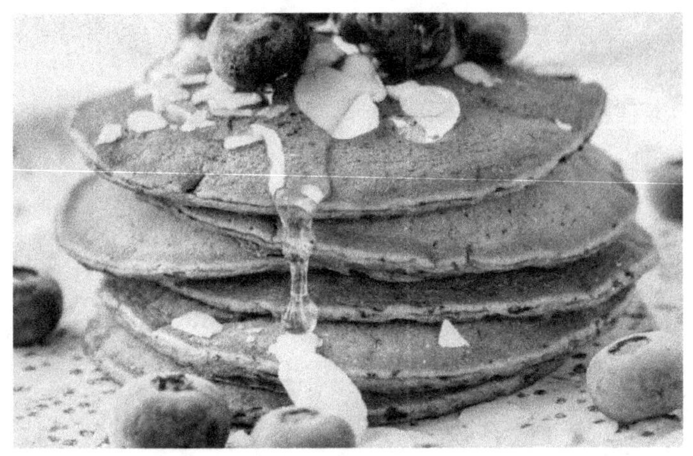

Sweet Potato Breakfast Bowl:

<u>Ingredients</u>: Roasted sweet potato, Greek yogurt, granola, honey.

<u>Instructions</u>:

- Add Greek yogurt and granola as toppings to roasted sweet potato.
- Sprinkle some honey over the meal.
- Serve and enjoy!

<u>Prep Time</u>: 30 minutes (including roasting time)

<u>Nutritional Information</u>: Fiber, protein, and vitamins.

Egg and Vegetable Breakfast Burrito:

<u>Ingredients</u>: Whole grain tortilla, scrambled eggs, bell peppers, black beans, salsa.

<u>Instructions</u>:

- Stuff the tortilla with salsa, black beans, bell peppers, and scrambled eggs.
- Serve and enjoy!

<u>Prep Time</u>: 15 minutes

<u>Nutritional Information</u>: Protein, fiber, and antioxidants.

Cinnamon Apple Quinoa Bowl:

<u>Ingredients</u>: Quinoa, cinnamon, apple slices, almond butter.

<u>Instructions</u>:

- Cook the quinoa with cinnamon
- Serve it with apple slices and almond butter as toppings.

<u>Prep Time</u>: 20 minutes

<u>Nutritional Information</u>: Fiber, antioxidants, and healthy fats.

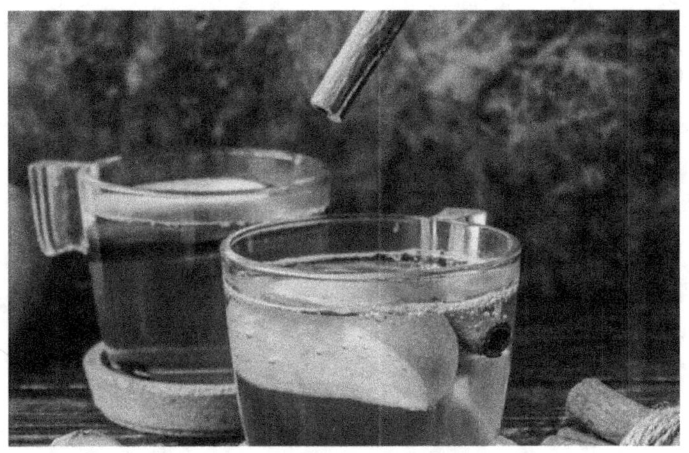

Spinach and Feta Omelet:

<u>Ingredients</u>: Eggs, spinach, feta cheese, cherry tomatoes.

<u>Instructions</u>:

- Beat the eggs and then add them to a pan along with cherry tomatoes, feta, and spinach.
- Stir to form an omelet.

<u>Prep Time</u>: 10 minutes

<u>Nutritional Information</u>: Protein, iron, and vitamins.

Blueberry Almond Overnight Oats:

<u>Ingredients</u>: Rolled oats, almond milk, blueberries, almond slices.

<u>Instructions</u>:

- Mix oats with almond milk
- Add blueberries and layer with almond slices.
- Allow to settle overnight.

<u>Prep Time</u>: 5 minutes (plus soaking time)

<u>Nutritional Information</u>: Fiber, antioxidants, and healthy fats.

Tomato and Avocado Breakfast Salad:

<u>Ingredients</u>: Cherry tomatoes, avocado, cucumber, red onion, olive oil.

<u>Instructions</u>:

- Mix cherry tomatoes, avocado, cucumber, and red onion.
- Spritz with olive oil.
- Serve and enjoy!

<u>Prep Time</u>: 10 minutes

<u>Nutritional Information</u>: Healthy fats, vitamins, and antioxidants.

Zucchini and Tomato Breakfast Bake:

<u>Ingredients</u>: Zucchini, cherry tomatoes, eggs, mozzarella cheese.

<u>Instructions</u>:

- Arrange the cherry tomatoes and sliced zucchini in a baking dish.
- Spoon whisked eggs onto it
- Sprinkle mozzarella on top.
- Bake for a while.

<u>Prep Time</u>: 25 minutes

<u>Nutritional Information</u>: Protein, vitamin C, and calcium.

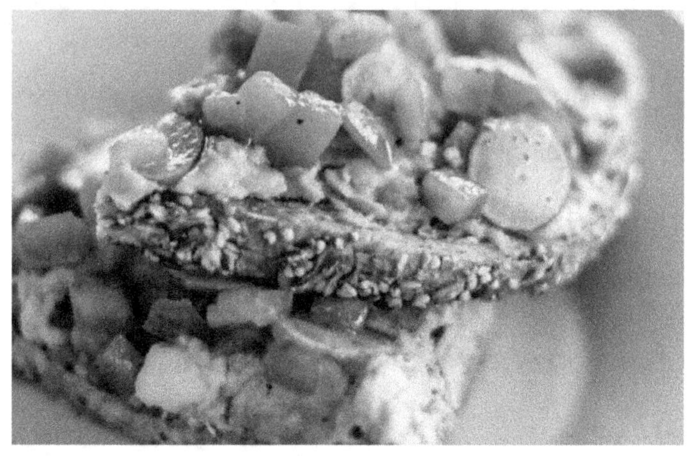

Orange and Ginger Chia Pudding:

<u>Ingredients</u>: Chia seeds, almond milk, orange zest, fresh ginger.

<u>Instructions</u>: Combine chia seeds and almond milk.

- Mix with grated ginger and orange zest and allow to set.

<u>Prep Time</u>: 10 minutes (plus soaking time)

<u>Nutritional Information</u>: Antioxidants, fiber, and anti-inflammatory properties.

CHAPTER 3: LUNCH RECIPE

Lentil and Vegetable Soup:

Ingredients: Lentils, carrots, celery, onions, vegetable broth, turmeric.

Instructions:

- Prepare the broth with turmeric.
- Cook lentils and vegetables in it.

Prep Time: 30 minutes

Nutritional Information: Fiber, protein, and anti-inflammatory spices.

Grilled Chicken and Quinoa Bowl:

Ingredients: Grilled chicken breast, quinoa, roasted vegetables, olive oil.

Instructions:

- Mix grilled chicken, quinoa, and veggies.
- Spritz with olive oil

Prep Time: 25 minutes

<u>Nutritional Information</u>: Protein, fiber, and essential vitamins.

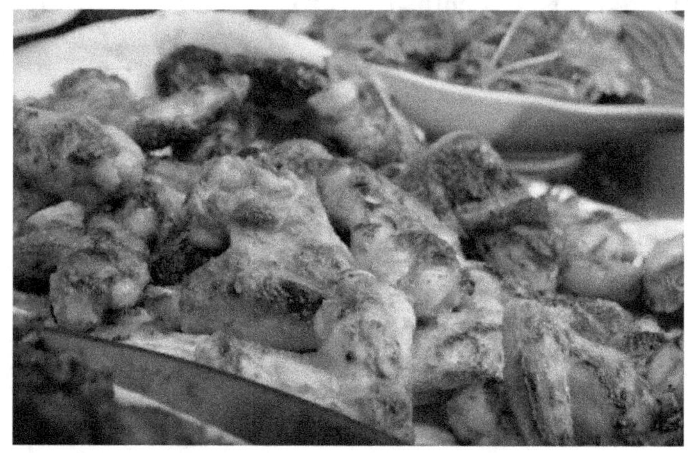

Mushroom and Spinach Stuffed Bell Peppers:

<u>Ingredients</u>: Bell peppers, mushrooms, spinach, quinoa, feta cheese.

<u>Instructions</u>:

- Sauté mushrooms and spinach
- Add quinoa and feta

- Stuff the bell peppers with the mixture and bake.

Prep Time: 35 minutes

Nutritional Information: Fiber, vitamins, and anti-inflammatory properties.

Sweet Potato and Chickpea Curry:

Ingredients: Sweet potatoes, chickpeas, coconut milk, curry spices.

Instructions:

- Simmer chickpeas and sweet potatoes with curry spices in coconut milk.
- Serve and enjoy.

Prep Time: 40 minutes

Nutritional Information: Protein, fiber and anti-inflammatory spices.

Tuna and Avocado Lettuce Wraps:

Ingredients: Canned tuna, avocado, lettuce leaves, cherry tomatoes.

<u>Instructions</u>:

- Combine avocado and tuna.
- Scoop onto lettuce leaves.
- Top with tomatoes and serve.

<u>Prep Time</u>: 15 minutes

<u>Nutritional Information</u>: Omega-3 fatty acids, vitamins, and minerals.

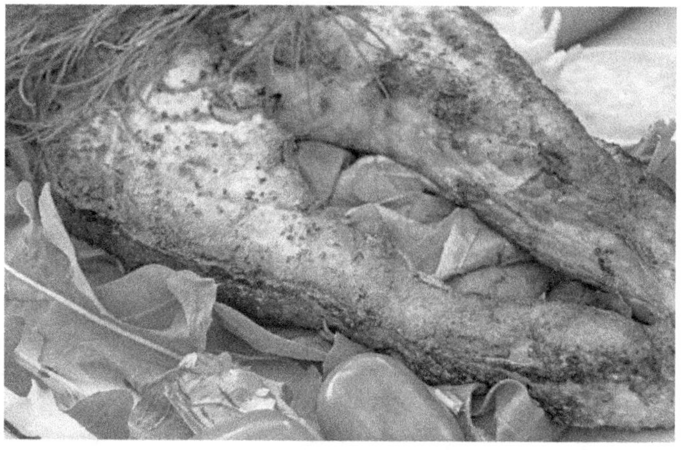

Broccoli and Almond Stir-Fry:

<u>Ingredients</u>: Broccoli, almonds, tofu, soy sauce, ginger.

<u>Instructions</u>:

- Prepare soy sauce with ginger.
- Stir-fry broccoli, almonds, and tofu in the soy sauce with ginger.

<u>Prep Time</u>: 25 minutes

<u>Nutritional Information</u>: Vitamins, protein, and healthy fats.

Chickpea and Spinach Stew:

<u>Ingredients</u>: Chickpeas, spinach, tomatoes, onions, garlic, cumin.

<u>Instructions</u>:

- Cook chickpeas, spinach, tomatoes, onions, and garlic.
- Add cumin and serve.

<u>Prep Time</u>: 30 minutes

<u>Nutritional Information</u>: Protein, iron, and anti-inflammatory properties.

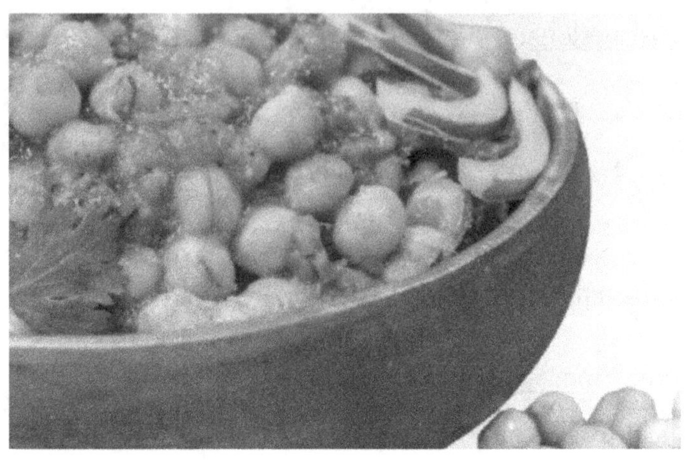

Cauliflower and Lentil Tacos:

<u>Ingredients</u>: Cauliflower, lentils, taco shells, salsa, guacamole.

<u>Instructions</u>:

- Roast the cauliflower.
- Prepare the lentils.
- Stuff the taco shells.
- Add guacamole and salsa as toppings.

<u>Prep Time</u>: 30 minutes

<u>Nutritional Information</u>: Protein, fiber, and anti-inflammatory spices.

Turmeric Chicken and Vegetable Skewers:

Ingredients: Chicken breast, bell peppers, zucchini, cherry tomatoes, turmeric.

Instructions:

- Put the chicken and vegetables on skewers.
- Grill and season with turmeric.

Prep Time: 30 minutes

Nutritional Information: Protein, antioxidants, and anti-inflammatory properties.

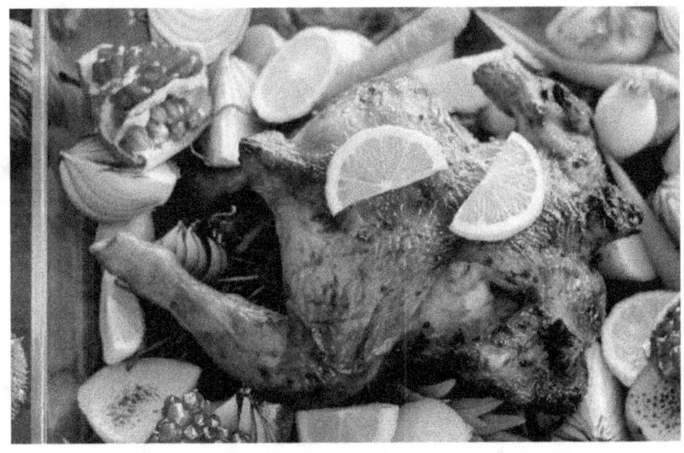

Wild Rice and Cranberry Salad:

<u>Ingredients</u>: Wild rice, dried cranberries, pecans, green onions, vinaigrette.

<u>Instructions</u>:

- Mix cooked wild rice, pecans, and vinaigrette, then stir

<u>Prep Time</u>: 25 minutes

<u>Nutritional Information</u>: Fiber, antioxidants, and essential nutrients.

Sesame Ginger Tofu Stir-Fry:

<u>Ingredients</u>: Tofu, broccoli, bell peppers, snap peas, sesame ginger sauce.

<u>Instructions</u>:

- Cook the tofu and vegetables in sesame ginger sauce.

<u>Prep Time</u>: 25 minutes

<u>Nutritional Information</u>: Protein, vitamins, and anti-inflammatory spices.

Zucchini Noodles with Pesto:

<u>Ingredients</u>: Zucchini noodles, cherry tomatoes, pine nuts, basil pesto.

<u>Instructions</u>:

- Sauté the zucchini noodles and then combine them with pesto, pine nuts, and tomatoes.

<u>Prep Time</u>: 15 minutes

<u>Nutritional Information</u>: Low-carb, vitamins, and healthy fats.

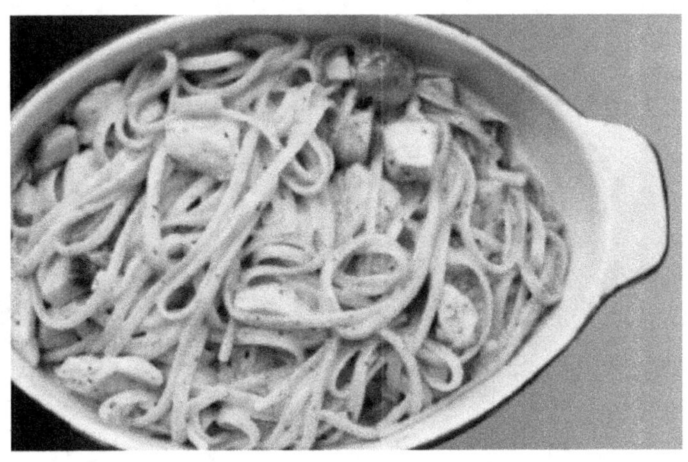

Cabbage and Carrot Slaw with Ginger Dressing:

<u>Ingredients</u>: Shredded cabbage, grated carrots, sesame seeds, ginger dressing.

<u>Instructions</u>: Combine carrots and cabbage with ginger dressing and sesame seeds.

<u>Prep Time</u>: 15 minutes

<u>Nutritional Information</u>: Vitamins, antioxidants, and anti-inflammatory properties.

Cilantro Lime Chicken Bowl:

<u>Ingredients</u>: Grilled chicken, brown rice, black beans, corn, cilantro lime dressing.

<u>Instructions</u>:

- Combine the rice, beans, corn, and grilled chicken.
- Pour on some cilantro lime vinaigrette.

<u>Prep Time</u>: 30 minutes

<u>Nutritional Information</u>: Protein, fiber, and vitamins.

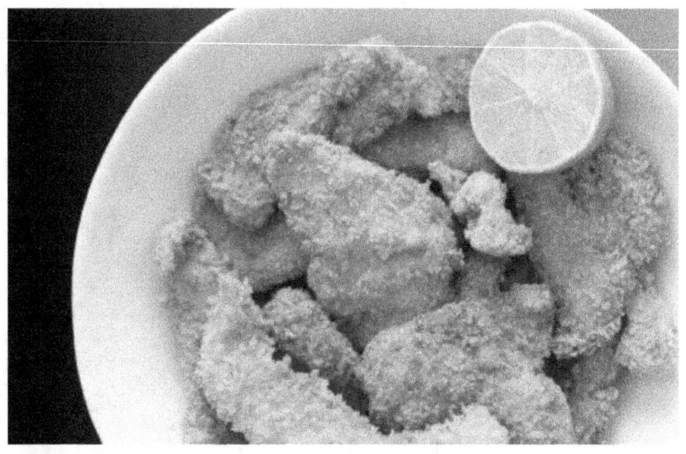

Brussels Sprouts and Quinoa Pilaf:

<u>Ingredients</u>: Brussels sprouts, quinoa, cranberries, pecans, balsamic vinaigrette.

<u>Instructions</u>:

- Roast Brussels sprouts
- Stir in pecans, cranberries, and cooked quinoa.
- Pour balsamic vinaigrette over.

<u>Prep Time</u>: 30 minutes

<u>Nutritional Information</u>: Fiber, antioxidants, and essential nutrients.

Cucumber and Avocado Gazpacho:

<u>Ingredients</u>: Cucumbers, avocados, tomatoes, bell peppers, cilantro.

<u>Instructions</u>:

- Blend cucumbers, avocados, cilantro, tomatoes, and peppers
- Refrigerate before serving.

<u>Prep Time</u>: 15 minutes

<u>Nutritional Information</u>: Hydrating, vitamins, and healthy fats.

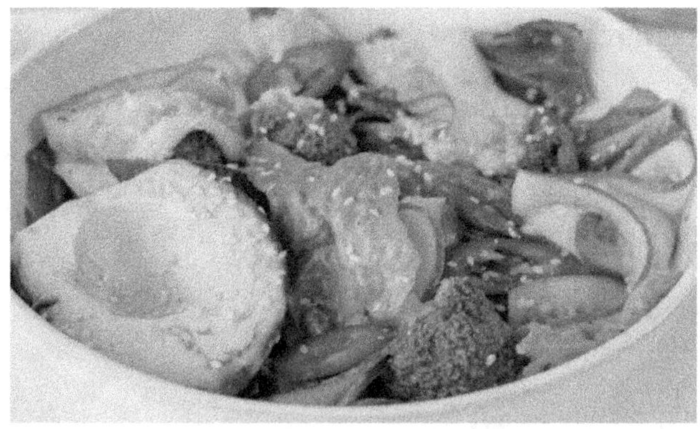

CHAPTER 4: DINNER RECIPES

Salmon with Turmeric and Lemon:

<u>Ingredients</u>: Salmon fillet, turmeric, lemon, olive oil.

<u>Instructions</u>:

- Add turmeric to the salmon and sprinkle it with lemon
- Bake it until it's flaky

<u>Prep Time</u>: 20 minutes

<u>Nutritional Information</u>: Omega-3 fatty acids, anti-inflammatory turmeric, and vitamin C.

Quinoa Stuffed Bell Peppers:

<u>Ingredients</u>: Quinoa, bell peppers, black beans, tomatoes.

Instructions: Stuff cooked quinoa mixture inside peppers along with black beans and tomatoes, then bake.

Prep Time: 30 minutes

Nutritional Information: Protein, fiber and antioxidants

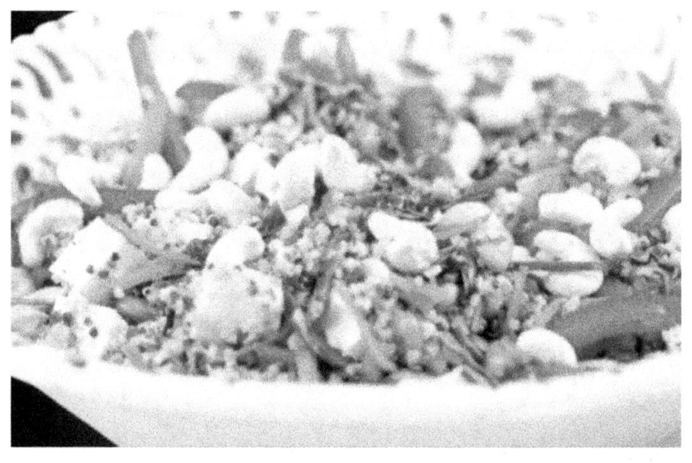

Turmeric and Garlic Shrimp Stir-Fry:

Ingredients: Shrimp, turmeric, garlic, vegetables, soy sauce.

<u>Instructions</u>:

- Sauté the shrimp with turmeric and garlic
- Add the veggies
- Whisk in the soy sauce, then serve.

<u>Prep Time</u>: 15 minutes

<u>Nutritional Information</u>: Protein, anti-inflammatory spices, and vitamins.

Mushroom and Spinach Quiche:

<u>Ingredients</u>: Pie crust, eggs, mushrooms, spinach, cheese.

<u>Instructions</u>:

- Whisk the eggs, spinach, and sautéed mushrooms
- Pour into pie crust and bake.

<u>Prep Time</u>: 40 minutes

<u>Nutritional Information</u>: Protein, iron, and vitamins.

Lemon Herb Baked Chicken:

<u>Ingredients</u>: Chicken breasts, lemon, herbs, olive oil.

<u>Instructions</u>:

- Marinate chicken with olive oil, lemon juice, and herbs.
- Bake until properly cooked.

<u>Prep Time</u>: 25 minutes

<u>Nutritional Information</u>: Lean protein, vitamin C, and anti-inflammatory herbs.

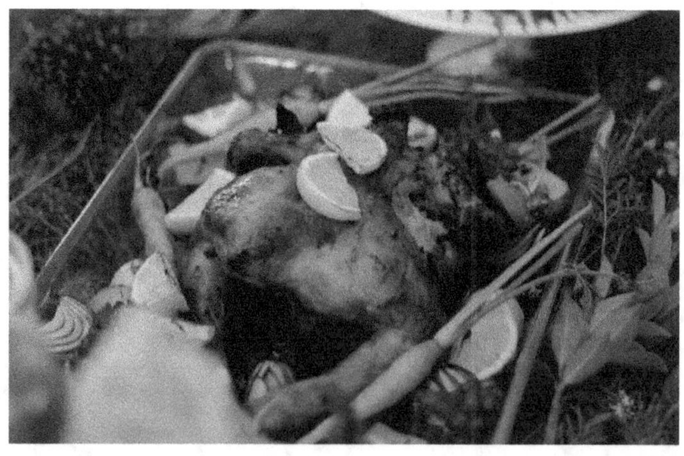

Vegetarian Lentil Soup:

Ingredients: Lentils, vegetables, vegetable broth, turmeric.

Instructions:

- Simmer lentils and vegetables in broth.
- Season with turmeric then cook.
- Serve and enjoy.

Prep Time: 30 minutes

Nutritional Information: Protein, fiber, and anti-inflammatory properties.

Cauliflower and Chickpea Curry:

Ingredients: Cauliflower, chickpeas, tomatoes, coconut milk.

Instructions:

- Sauté cauliflower and chickpeas in a tomato-and-coconut-milk curry sauce.
- Serve and enjoy!

Prep Time: 35 minutes

Nutritional Information: Fiber, protein, and anti-inflammatory spices.

Spinach and Feta Stuffed Chicken Breast:

Ingredients: Chicken breasts, spinach, feta, garlic.

Instructions:

- Stuff chicken breasts with feta, sautéed spinach, and garlic, then bake.

Prep Time: 30 minutes

Nutritional Information: Protein, iron, and calcium.

Pesto Zucchini Noodles with Grilled Chicken:

Ingredients: Zucchini, chicken breasts, pesto sauce.

Instructions:

- Grill the chicken
- Spiralize the zucchini
- Stir with pesto, and serve.

<u>Prep Time</u>: 25 minutes

<u>Nutritional Information</u>: Lean protein, vitamins, and healthy fats.

Broccoli and Almond Stir-Fry:

<u>Ingredients</u>: Broccoli, almonds, garlic, soy sauce.

<u>Instructions</u>:

- Cook broccoli and almonds with garlic.
- Finish with a dash of soy sauce.

<u>Prep Time</u>: 15 minutes

<u>Nutritional Information</u>: Fiber, antioxidants, and healthy fats.

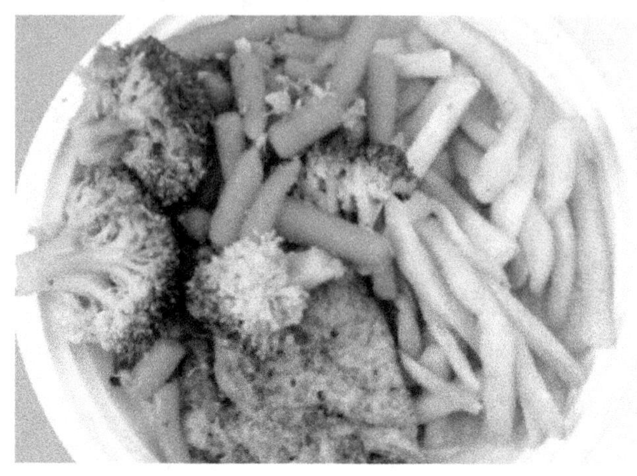

Miso Glazed Salmon:

Ingredients: Salmon fillet, miso paste, honey, soy sauce.

Instructions: Coat fish with miso, honey, and soy sauce and broil until caramelized.

Prep Time: 20 minutes

Nutritional Information: Omega-3 fatty acids, probiotics from miso, and protein.

Cabbage and Turmeric Sauté:

Ingredients: Cabbage, turmeric, onions, olive oil.

Instructions:

- Using olive oil, sauté cabbage and onions with turmeric till soft.

Prep Time: 15 minutes

Nutritional Information: Fiber, vitamins and Anti-inflammatory turmeric.

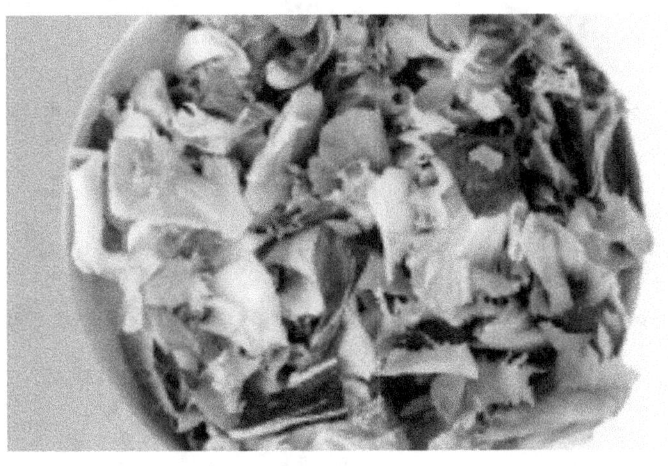

Garlic Lemon Herb Roasted Vegetables:

Ingredients: Assorted vegetables, garlic, lemon, herbs.

Instructions:

- Toss the vegetables with the garlic, lemon, and herbs and roast until golden brown.

Prep Time: 30 minutes

Nutritional Information: Fiber, vitamins, and antioxidants.

Chicken and Vegetable Skewers:

Ingredients: Chicken breast, bell peppers, cherry tomatoes, olive oil.

Instructions:

- Thread the chicken and vegetables onto the skewers.
- Drizzle with olive oil and cook.
- Serve and enjoy!

Prep Time: 25 minutes

Nutritional Information: Protein, vitamins, and healthy fats.

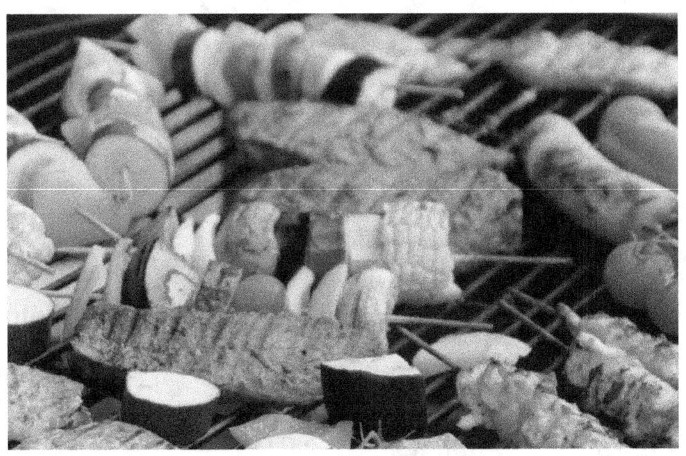

Lemon Garlic Shrimp Pasta:

Ingredients: Whole wheat pasta, shrimp, lemon, garlic, olive oil.

Instructions:

- Cook the pasta.
- Sauté shrimp with lemon and garlic.
- Toss with pasta.

Prep Time: 20 minutes

Nutritional Information: Protein, whole grains, and heart-healthy fats.

Baked Cod with Tomato Basil Relish:

Ingredients: Cod fillet, tomatoes, basil, olive oil.

Instructions:

- Bake cod.
- Add diced tomatoes and basil drizzled with olive oil as toppings.

Prep Time: 25 minutes

Nutritional Information: Protein, vitamins, and healthy fats.

Kale and Walnut Pesto Pasta:

Ingredients: Whole wheat pasta, kale, walnuts, garlic, olive oil.

Instructions:

- To prepare pesto, blend kale, walnuts, garlic, and olive oil.
- Mix with pasta.
- Serve and enjoy.

Prep Time: 20 minutes

<u>Nutritional Information</u>: Fiber, omega-3 fatty acids, and vitamins.

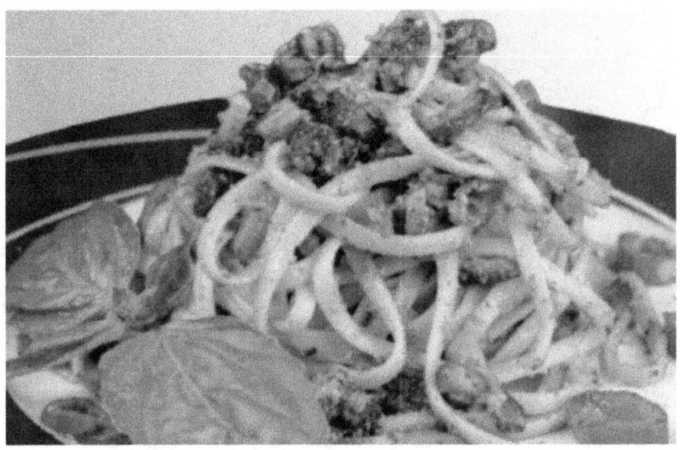

Mediterranean Chickpea Salad:

<u>Ingredients</u>: Chickpeas, cucumber, tomatoes, feta cheese, olives.

<u>Instructions</u>:

- Mix chickpeas, cucumber, tomatoes, feta, and olives in a bowl.
- Sprinkle the mixture with olive oil.
- Serve and enjoy.

<u>Prep Time</u>: 15 minutes

<u>Nutritional Information</u>: Protein, fiber, and healthy fats.

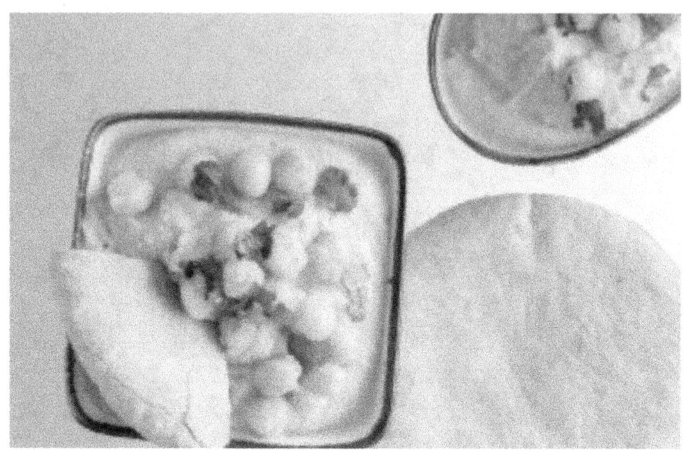

Lemon Dill Baked Salmon:

<u>Ingredients</u>: Salmon fillet, lemon, dill, olive oil.

<u>Instructions</u>:

- Marinate the salmon in lemon, dill, and olive oil
- Afterwards, bake until it is flaky.

<u>Prep Time</u>: 20 minutes

<u>Nutritional Information</u>: Omega-3 fatty acids, vitamin C, and anti-inflammatory herbs.

CHAPTER 5: SALAD RECIPES

Beet and Walnut Salad:

<u>Ingredients</u>: Beets, arugula, walnuts, goat cheese.

<u>Instructions</u>:

- Mix roasted beets, arugula, walnuts, and crumbled goat cheese.

<u>Prep Time</u>: 25 minutes

<u>Nutritional Information</u>: Antioxidants, omega-3s, and calcium.

Cauliflower and Chickpea Salad:

<u>Ingredients</u>: Roasted cauliflower, chickpeas, mint and cucumber.

<u>Instructions</u>:

- Mix the roasted cauliflower, chickpeas, diced cucumber, and chopped mint in a mixing bowl.

- Serve and enjoy!

<u>Prep Time</u>: 30 minutes

<u>Nutritional Information</u>: Fiber, protein, and anti-inflammatory properties.

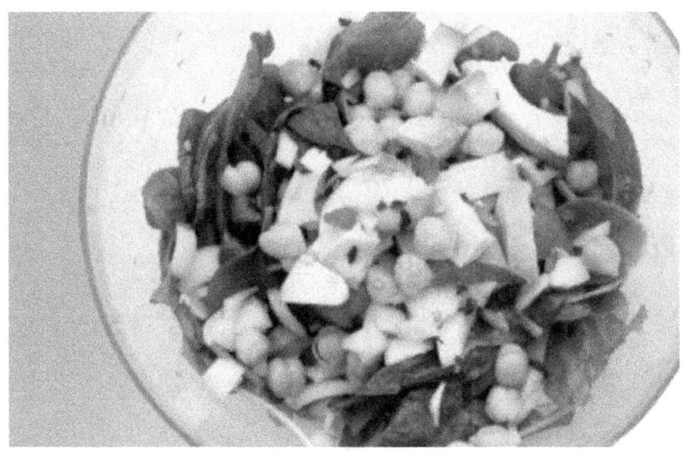

Arugula and Pear Salad:

<u>Ingredients</u>: Arugula, pears, pecans, blue cheese.

<u>Instructions</u>:

- Mix arugula, sliced pears, toasted walnuts, and crumbled blue cheese in a salad bowl.
- Serve in a plate and enjoy!

Prep Time: 15 minutes

Nutritional Information: Vitamin K, fiber, and calcium.

Tomato Basil Mozzarella Salad:

Ingredients: Cherry tomatoes, fresh mozzarella, basil, balsamic glaze.

Instructions:

- Mix the half tomatoes, mozzarella balls, and torn basil in a mixing bowl.
- Drizzle the balsamic glaze over the top.
- Dish into plates and enjoy!

Prep Time: 10 minutes

Nutritional Information: Calcium, antioxidants, and heart-healthy fats.

Greek Quinoa Salad:

Ingredients: Quinoa, cherry tomatoes, cucumber, olives, feta.

Instructions:

- Mix cooked quinoa, tomatoes, cucumber, olives, and crumbled feta in a mixing bowl.
- Drizzle with olive oil.

<u>Prep Time</u>: 20 minutes

<u>Nutritional Information</u>: Protein, calcium, and healthy fats.

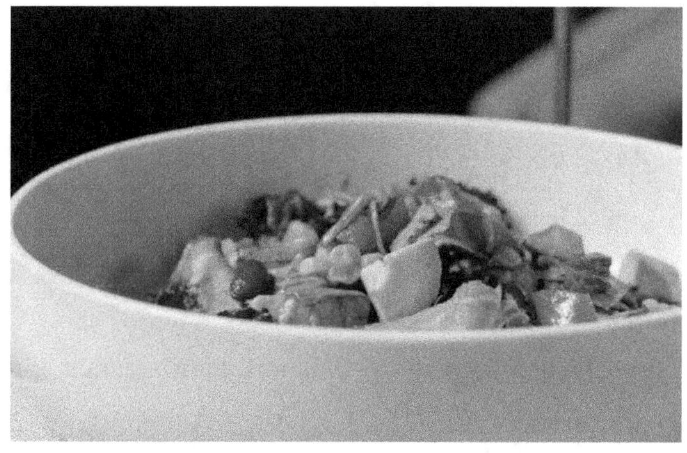

Broccoli and Cranberry Salad:

<u>Ingredients</u>: Broccoli, dried cranberries, sunflower seeds.

<u>Instructions</u>:

- Toss broccoli with cranberries and sunflower seeds after steaming.
- Add dressing by drizzling honey mustard dressing over it.

Prep Time: 15 minutes

Nutritional Information: Fiber, antioxidants, and vitamin C.

Pesto Caprese Salad:

Ingredients: Tomatoes, fresh mozzarella, basil, pesto.

Instructions:

- Arrange sliced tomatoes, mozzarella, and basil on a platter.
- Drizzle pesto on top.
- Serve on a plate and enjoy!

Prep Time: 10 minutes

Nutritional Information: Antioxidants, calcium, and healthy fats.

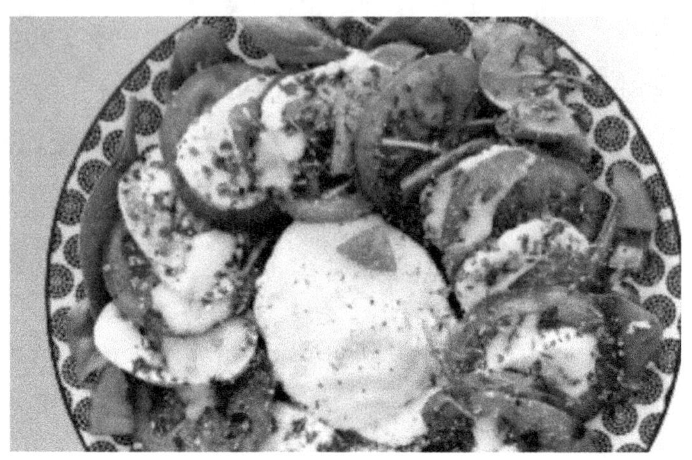

Spinach and Walnut Salad:

<u>Ingredients</u>: Baby spinach, walnuts, apples, feta.

<u>Instructions</u>:

- Mix spinach, apples, walnuts, and crumbled feta in a mixing bowl.
- Add vinaigrette to the mixture.
- Serve and enjoy!

<u>Prep Time</u>: 15 minutes

<u>Nutritional Information</u>: Iron, omega-3s, and calcium.

Cucumber and Radish Salad:

<u>Ingredients</u>: Cucumber, radishes, Greek yogurt, dill.

<u>Instructions</u>:

- Slice cucumber and radishes and combine with Greek yogurt and dill.
- Dish on a plate and enjoy.

<u>Prep Time</u>: 10 minutes

<u>Nutritional Information</u>: Hydrating, probiotics, and antioxidants.

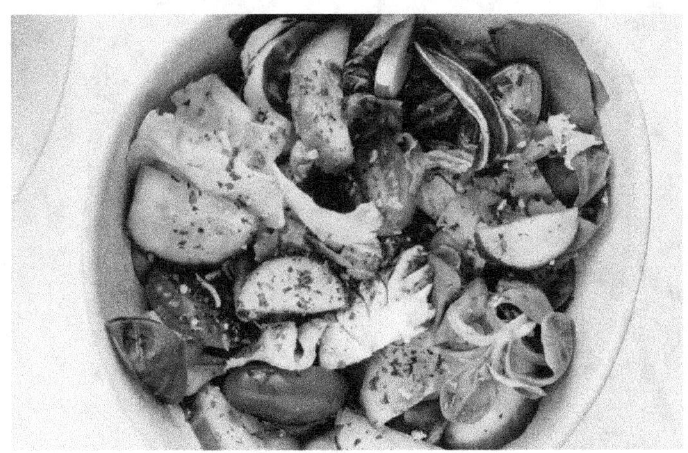

Pear and Walnut Salad:

Ingredients: Mixed greens, pears, walnuts, blue cheese.

Instructions:

- Toss together the mixed greens, sliced pears, walnuts, and crumbled blue cheese.
- Drizzle with balsamic vinaigrette and serve.

Prep Time: 15 minutes

Nutritional Information: Vitamin K, omega-3s, and calcium.

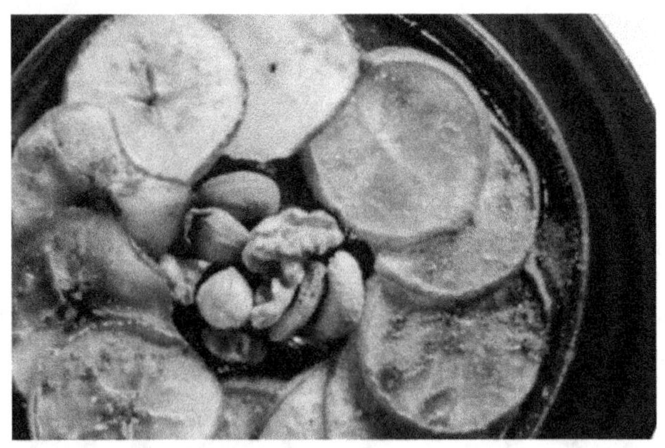

CHAPTER 6: SNACKS RECIPES

Turmeric Roasted Chickpeas:

Ingredients: Chickpeas, olive oil, turmeric, cumin, salt.

Instructions:

- Roast chickpeas in olive oil and seasonings till golden and crunchy.
- Serve as it is ready to eat.

Prep Time: 30 minutes

Nutritional Information: Protein, fiber, and anti-inflammatory turmeric.

Almond Butter and Banana Rice Cakes:

Ingredients: Rice cakes, almond butter, banana slices.

- Make rice cakes.
- Top with almond butter and banana slices.

<u>Prep Time</u>: 5 minutes

<u>Nutritional Information</u>: Healthy fats, potassium, and protein.

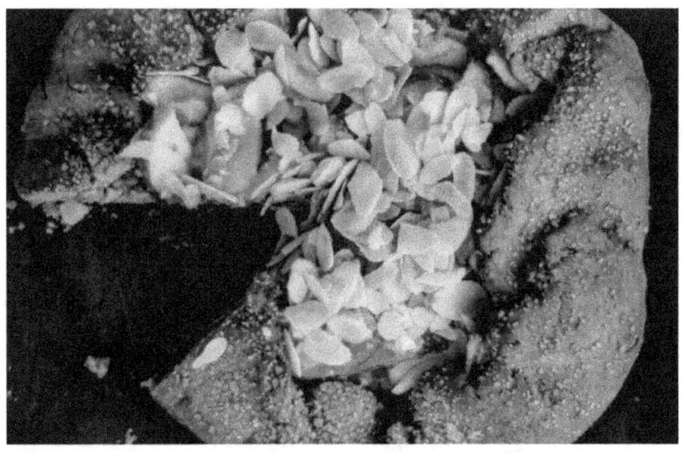

Turmeric Spiced Nuts:

<u>Ingredients</u>: Mixed nuts, olive oil, turmeric, black pepper.

Instructions:

- Toss the nuts with the olive oil, turmeric, and black pepper before baking until aromatic

Prep Time: 15 minutes

Nutritional Information: Omega-3s, protein, and anti-inflammatory turmeric.

Sliced Apple with Almond Butter:

Ingredients: Apples, almond butter, chia seeds.

Instructions:

- Dip apples in almond butter and top with chia seeds.

Prep Time: 5 minutes

Nutritional Information: Fiber, healthy fats, and omega-3s.

Kale Chips:

Ingredients: Kale leaves, olive oil, nutritional yeast.

Instructions:

- Rub greens with olive oil, then sprinkle with nutritional yeast and bake till crisp.

Prep Time: 20 minutes

Nutritional Information: Vitamin K, fiber, and antioxidants.

Chia Pudding with Mango:

Ingredients: Chia seeds, almond milk, mango, honey.

Instructions:

- Refrigerate chia seeds and almond milk, then top with diced mango
- Drizzle with honey.

Prep Time: 5 minutes (plus overnight chilling)

Nutritional Information: Omega-3s, fiber, and vitamins.

Carrot and Hummus Dip:

Ingredients: Carrot sticks, hummus.

Instructions:

- Dip carrot sticks in hummus for a protein-packed snack.

<u>Prep Time</u>: 5 minutes

<u>Nutritional Information</u>: Beta-carotene, fiber, and protein.

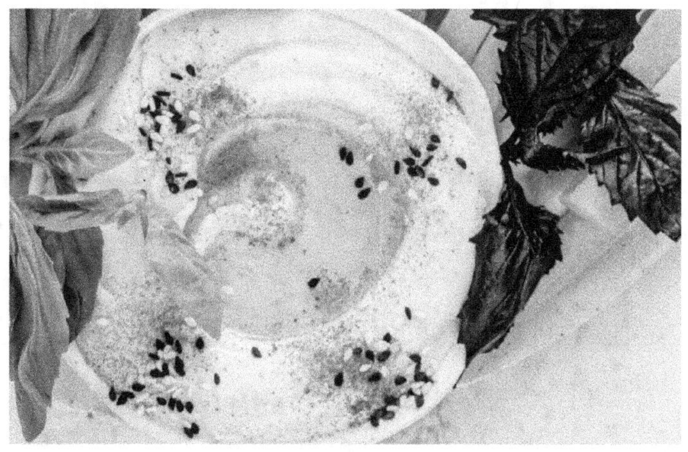

Caprese Skewers:

<u>Ingredients</u>: Cherry tomatoes, fresh mozzarella, basil, balsamic glaze.

<u>Instructions</u>: Drizzle with balsamic glaze after threading tomatoes, mozzarella, and basil onto skewers.

<u>Prep Time</u>: 10 minutes

<u>Nutritional Information</u>: Calcium, antioxidants, and heart-healthy fats.

Pumpkin Seeds with Cinnamon:

Ingredients: Pumpkin seeds, olive oil, cinnamon.

<u>Instructions</u>:

- Roast pumpkin seeds in olive oil and cinnamon till crispy.

<u>Prep Time</u>: 15 minutes

<u>Nutritional Information</u>: Protein, fiber, and anti-inflammatory cinnamon.

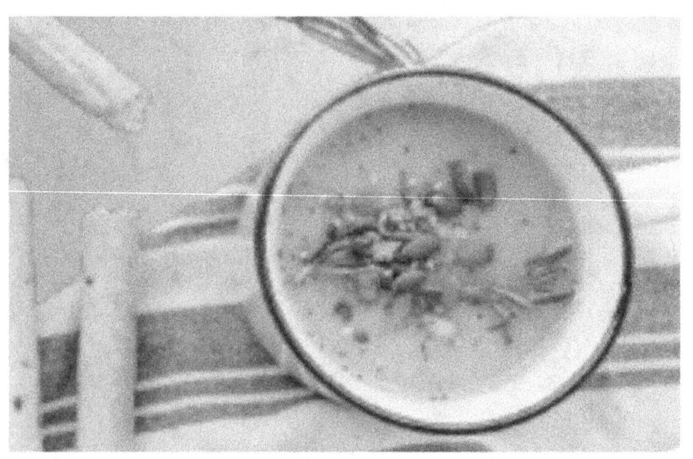

Coconut and Berry Energy Bites:

<u>Ingredients</u>: Dates, coconut flakes, mixed berries.

<u>Instructions</u>:

- Blend dates, coconut flakes, and berries.
- Shape into energy bits and serve

<u>Prep Time</u>: 15 minutes

<u>Nutritional Information</u>: Natural sweetness, fiber, and vitamins.

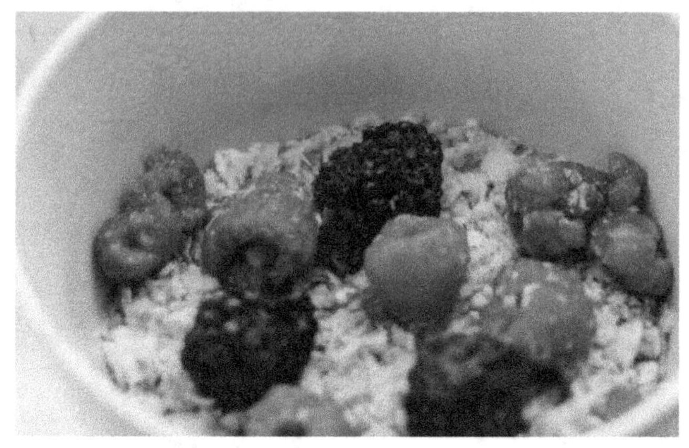

Mango and Chili Lime Dip:

<u>Ingredients</u>: Mango, lime juice, chili powder.

<u>Instructions</u>:

- For a zesty and delicious dip, dice mango and combine with lime juice and a sprinkle of chili powder.

<u>Prep Time</u>: 10 minutes

<u>Nutritional Information</u>: Vitamin C, antioxidants, and a touch of spice.

CHAPTER 7: SMOTHIE RECIPES

Green Goddess Smoothie:

<u>Ingredients</u>: Spinach, banana, pineapple, Greek yogurt.

<u>Instructions</u>:

- Blend spinach, banana, pineapple, and Greek yogurt until you get a smooth feel.
- Serve and enjoy!

<u>Prep Time</u>: 5 minutes

<u>Nutritional Information</u>: Rich in antioxidants, fiber, and probiotics.

Turmeric Mango Bliss:

<u>Ingredients</u>: Mango, turmeric, coconut milk, chia seeds.

<u>Instructions</u>:

- Blend mango, turmeric, coconut milk, and chia seeds until it is creamy.
- Serve and enjoy!

<u>Prep Time</u>: 7 minutes

<u>Nutritional Information</u>: Anti-inflammatory, high in vitamins, and omega-3 fatty acids.

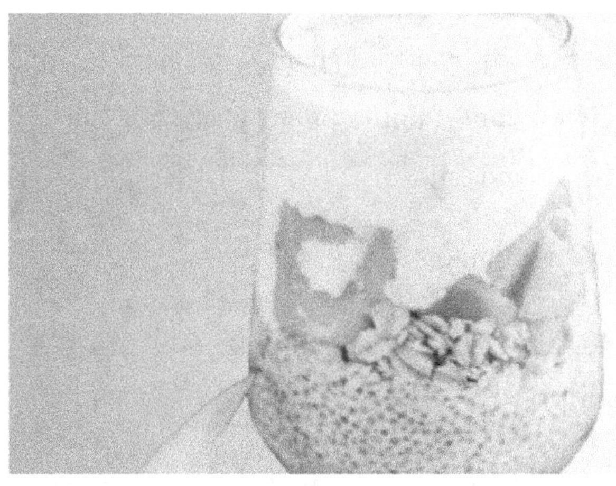

Pineapple Ginger Zing:

<u>Ingredients</u>: Pineapple, ginger, cucumber, coconut water.

Instructions: For a refreshing zing, blend pineapple, ginger, cucumber, and coconut water.

Prep Time: 6 minutes

Nutritional Information: anti-inflammatory, hydrating and rich in vitamins

Raspberry Avocado Revitalizer:

Ingredients: Raspberries, avocado, kale, almond milk.

Instructions:

- For a rejuvenating smoothie, blend raspberries, avocado, kale with almond milk.
- Enjoy the drink

Prep Time: 8 minutes

Nutritional Information: Omega-3 fatty acids, antioxidants, and vitamins.

Papaya Passion Twist:

Ingredients: Papaya, passion fruit, banana, coconut water.

Instructions:

- For a tropical twist, blend papaya, passion fruit, banana, and coconut water till it is smooth.
- Serve and enjoy.

Prep Time: 6 minutes

Nutritional Information: Vitamin C, fiber, and hydration.

Coconut Berry Bliss:

Ingredients: Mixed berries, coconut milk, chia seeds, honey.

Instructions:

- Blend berries, coconut milk, chia seeds, and honey until you get a smooth feel
- Serve and enjoy

Prep Time: 7 minutes

Nutritional Information: Antioxidants and omega-3 fatty acids

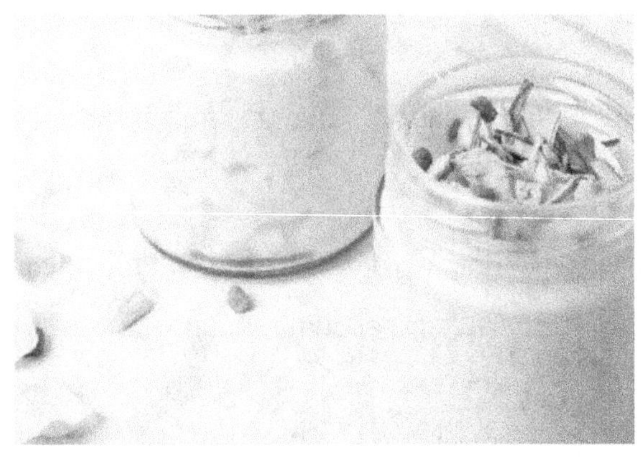

Peach Ginger Energy Elixir:

<u>Ingredients</u>: Peaches, ginger, Greek yogurt, almond milk.

<u>Instructions</u>:

- To make an energy-boosting elixir, blend peaches, ginger, Greek yogurt, with almond milk till you get a smooth feel.

<u>Prep Time</u>: 7 minutes

<u>Nutritional Information</u>: Antioxidants, probiotics, and natural energy.

Tropical Turmeric Tango:

<u>Ingredients</u>: Pineapple, mango, turmeric, coconut water.

<u>Instructions</u>: For a tropical tango, blend pineapple, mango, turmeric, and coconut water.

<u>Prep Time</u>: 6 minutes

<u>Nutritional Information</u>: Anti-inflammatory, vitamins, and hydration.

Chocolate Avocado Delight:

<u>Ingredients</u>: Avocado, cocoa powder, banana, almond milk.

<u>Instructions</u>:

- For a chocolatey treat, blend avocado, cocoa powder, banana with almond milk.

<u>Prep Time</u>: 6 minutes

<u>Nutritional Information</u>: Healthy fats, antioxidants, and potassium.

CHAPTER 8: BEVERAGES RECIPES

Anti-Inflammatory Iced Green Tea:

<u>Ingredients</u>: Green tea, turmeric, honey, lemon.

<u>Instructions</u>:

- Make green tea
- Add turmeric, honey, and lemon.
- Chill before serving over ice.

<u>Prep Time</u>: 10 minutes

<u>Nutritional Information</u>: Antioxidants, anti-inflammatory turmeric, and immune-boosting.

Raspberry Rosemary Sparkler:

<u>Ingredients</u>: Raspberries, rosemary, sparkling water, agave syrup.

<u>Instructions</u>:

- Muddle raspberries and rosemary in a strainer

- Add sparkling water

- Sweeten with agave.

<u>Prep Time</u>: 10 minutes

<u>Nutritional Information</u>: Antioxidants, herbs, and natural sweetness.

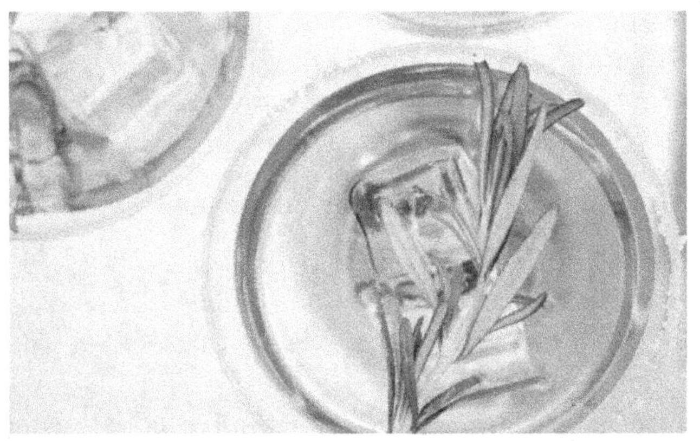

Detoxifying Green Juice:

<u>Ingredients</u>: Kale, cucumber, celery, lemon.

<u>Instructions</u>:

- Juice Kale, cucumber, celery, and lemon

- Serve over ice with a strainer.

<u>Prep Time</u>: 10 minutes

<u>Nutritional Information</u>: Detoxifying, vitamin C, and hydrating.

Carrot Ginger Elixir:

<u>Ingredients</u>: Carrots, ginger, orange, honey.

<u>Instructions</u>:

- Juice carrots, ginger, and orange.
- Stir with honey to taste.

<u>Prep Time</u>: 10 minutes

<u>Nutritional information</u>: Vitamin A, anti-inflammatory ginger, and immune-boosting.

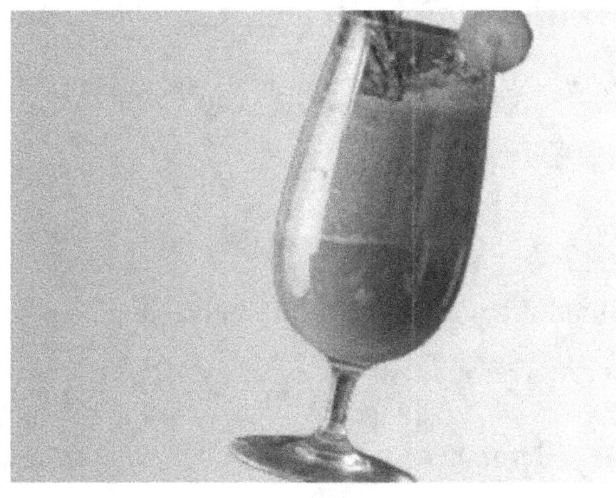

Blueberry Lavender Lemonade:

<u>Ingredients</u>: Blueberries, lavender, lemon, agave syrup.

<u>Instructions</u>:

- Blend blueberries, lavender, and lemon juice
- Chill after straining and sweetening with agave.

<u>Prep Time</u>: 15 minutes

<u>Nutritional Information</u>: Antioxidants, calming lavender, and vitamin C.

Minty Watermelon Refresher:

<u>Ingredients</u>: Watermelon, mint leaves, lime, sparkling water.

<u>Instructions</u>:

- Blend the watermelon, mint, and lime.
- Serve over ice with sparkling water.

<u>Prep Time</u>: 10 minutes

<u>Nutritional Information</u>: Hydrating, vitamins, and refreshing.

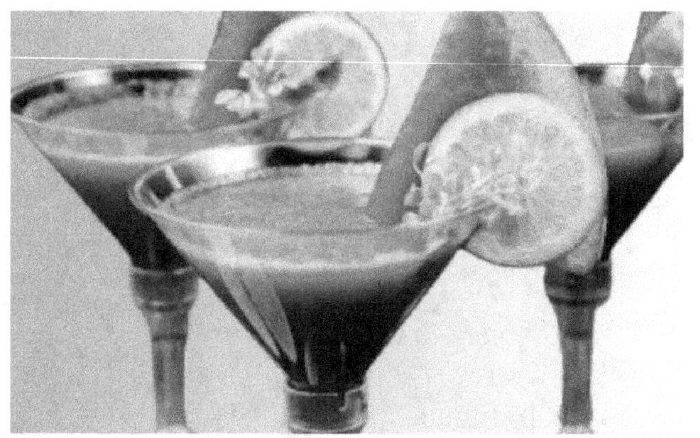

Pomegranate Basil Lemonade:

<u>Ingredients</u>: Pomegranate seeds, basil, lemon, honey.

<u>Instructions</u>:

- Blend pomegranate seeds, basil, and lemon juice
- Chill after straining and sweetening with honey.

<u>Prep Time</u>: 15 minutes

<u>Nutritional Information</u>: Antioxidants, anti-inflammatory basil, and vitamin C.

Ginger Lemon Honey Tea:

<u>Ingredients</u>: Fresh ginger, lemon, honey, hot water.

<u>Instructions</u>:

- Steep sliced ginger and lemon in hot water
- Add honey to taste.

<u>Prep Time</u>: 10 minutes

<u>Nutritional Information</u>: Anti-inflammatory ginger, vitamin C, and soothing.

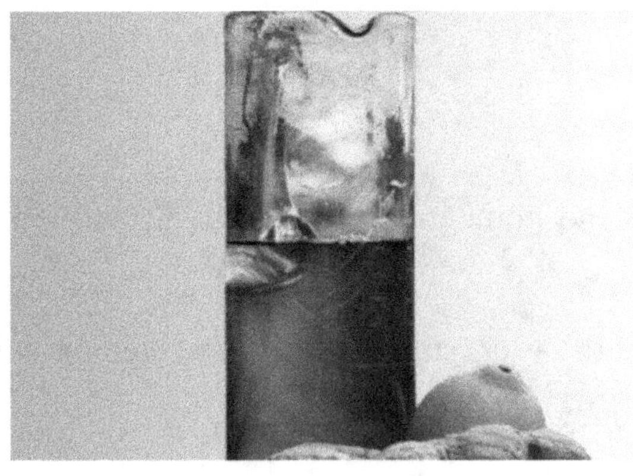

Chamomile Lavender Tea:

<u>Ingredients</u>: Chamomile tea bags, lavender, honey.

- Steep chamomile tea with lavender for 5 minutes
- Sweeten with honey and serve.

<u>Prep Time</u>: 5 minutes

<u>Nutritional Information</u>: Calming herbs, antioxidants, and soothing.

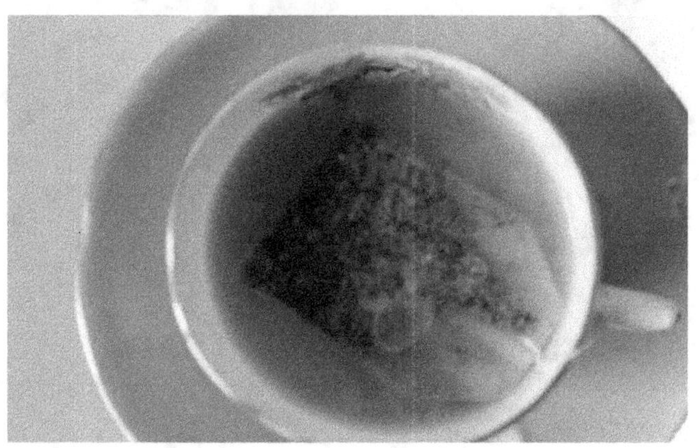

Cucumber Celery Green Juice:

<u>Ingredients</u>: Cucumber, celery, kale, lemon.

<u>Instructions</u>:

- Juice cucumber, celery, kale, and lemon
- Serve over ice with a strainer.

<u>Prep Time</u>: 10 minutes

<u>Nutritional Information</u>: Hydrating, vitamins, and detoxifying.

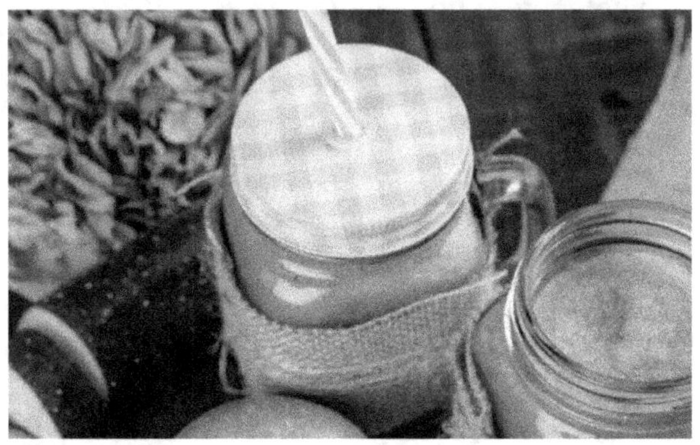

CHAPTER 9: MEAL PLAN

A thoughtful meal plan has been prepared to foster your well-being in this anti-inflammatory cookbook for beginners. Discover a symbiotic blend of colorful, nutrient-dense nutrients aimed at lowering inflammation in your body. Each recipe, from healthy breakfast options to filling feasts, is designed with simplicity and flavor in mind. With our carefully crafted meal plan, you can embrace a path toward greater health by making inflammation-fighting foods an accessible and delightful part of your regular kitchen experience.

Day 1:

Breakfast: Sweet Potato and Spinach Frittata

Snack: Mango and Chili Lime Dip

Lunch: Sesame Ginger Tofu Stir-Fry

Snack: Carrot and Hummus Dip

Dinner: Chicken and Vegetable Skewers

Day 2:

Breakfast: Oatmeal with Turmeric and Berries

Snack: Coconut Berry Bliss

Lunch: Lentil and Vegetable Soup

Snack: Almond Butter and Banana Rice Cakes

Dinner: Mediterranean Chickpea Salad

Day 3:

Breakfast: Mushroom and Spinach Breakfast Wrap

Snack: Cucumber Celery Green Juice

Lunch: Greek Quinoa Salad

Snack: Brussels Sprouts and Quinoa Pilaf

Dinner: Turmeric and Garlic Shrimp Stir-fry

Day 4:

Breakfast: Avocado Toast with Poached Egg

Snack: Blueberry Lavender Lemonade

Lunch: Tuna and Avocado Lettuce Wraps

Snack: Detoxifying Green Juice

Dinner: Baked Cod with Tomato Basil Relish

Day 5:

Breakfast: Chia Seed Pudding Parfait

Snack: Sliced Apple with Almond Butter

Lunch: Cauliflower and Chickpea Salad

Snack: Turmeric Spiced Nuts

Dinner: Lemon Herb Baked Chicken

Day 6:

Breakfast: Spinach and Feta Omelet

Snack: Coconut Berry Bliss

Lunch: Grilled Chicken and Quinoa Bowl

Snack: Arugula and Pear Salad

Dinner: Cabbage and Turmeric Sauté

Day 7:

Breakfast: Green Goddess Smoothie

Snack: Pineapple Ginger Zing:

Lunch: Sweet Potato and Chickpea Curry

Snack: Caprese Skewers

Dinner: Quinoa Stuffed Bell Peppers

Day 8:

Breakfast: Almond and Blueberry Protein Pancakes

Snack: Carrot and Hummus Dip

Lunch: Lentil and Vegetable Soup

Snack: Pomegranate Basil Lemonade

Dinner: Broccoli and Almond Stir-Fry

Day 9:

Breakfast: Blueberry Almond Overnight Oats

Snack: Sliced Apple with Almond Butter

Lunch: Chickpea and Spinach Stew

Snack: Peach Ginger Energy Elixir

Dinner: Kale and Walnut Pesto Pasta

Day 10:

Breakfast: Mushroom and Spinach Breakfast Wrap

Snack: Turmeric Spiced Nuts

Lunch: Cabbage and Carrot Slaw with Ginger Dressing

Snack: Cucumber and Radish Salad

Dinner: Lemon Garlic Shrimp Pasta

Day 11:

Breakfast: Quinoa Breakfast Porridge

Snack: Pear and Walnut Salad

Lunch: Chickpea and Spinach Stew

Snack: Kale Chips

Dinner: Baked Cod with Tomato Basil Relish

Day 12:

Breakfast: Almond and Blueberry Protein Pancakes

Snack: Tropical Turmeric Tango

Lunch: Turmeric Chicken and Vegetable Skewers

Snack: Carrot Ginger Elixir

Dinner: Lemon Dill Baked Salmon

Day 13:

Breakfast: Cauliflower and Kale Breakfast Hash

Snack: Green Goddess Smoothie

Lunch: Lentil and Vegetable Soup

Snack: Mango and Chili Lime Dip

Dinner: Pesto Zucchini Noodles with Grilled Chicken

Day 14:

Breakfast: Avocado Toast with Poached Egg

Snack: Almond Butter and Banana Rice Cakes

Lunch: Greek Quinoa Salad

Snack: Mango and Chili Lime Dip

Dinner: Kale and Walnut Pesto Pasta

Day 15:

Breakfast: Chia Seed Pudding Parfait

Snack: Blueberry Lavender Lemonade

Lunch: Turmeric Chicken and Vegetable Skewers

Snack: Cucumber Celery Green Juice

Dinner: Spinach and Feta Stuffed Chicken Breast

Day 16:

Breakfast: Tomato and Avocado Breakfast Salad

Snack: Coconut and Berry Energy Bites

Lunch: Cauliflower and Chickpea Salad

Snack: Chocolate Avocado Delight

Dinner: Lemon Garlic Shrimp Pasta

Day 17:

Breakfast: Green Tea Chia Pudding

Snack: Pineapple Ginger Zing

Lunch: Wild Rice and Cranberry Salad

Snack: Pumpkin Seeds with Cinnamon

Dinner: Lemon Herb Baked Chicken

Day 18:

Breakfast: Oatmeal with Turmeric and Berries

Snack: Pomegranate Basil Lemonade

Lunch: Cucumber and Avocado Gazpacho

Snack: Raspberry Avocado Revitalizer

Dinner: Baked Cod with Tomato Basil Relish

Day 19:

Breakfast: Egg and Vegetable Breakfast Burrito

Snack: Minty Watermelon Refresher

Lunch: Brussels Sprouts and Quinoa Pilaf

Snack: Ginger Lemon Honey Tea

Dinner: Miso Glazed Salmon

Day 20:

Breakfast: Mushroom and Spinach Breakfast Wrap

Snack: Raspberry Rosemary Sparkler

Lunch: Chickpea and Spinach Stew

Snack: Chia Pudding with Mango

Dinner: Mushroom and Spinach Quiche

Day 21:

Breakfast: Cinnamon Apple Quinoa Bowl

Snack: Carrot and Hummus Dip

Lunch: Mushroom and Spinach Stuffed Bell Peppers

Snack: Turmeric Roasted Chickpeas

Dinner: Turmeric and Garlic Shrimp Stir-Fry

Day 22:

Breakfast: Chocolate Avocado Delight

Snack: Kale Chips

Lunch: Tuna and Avocado Lettuce Wraps

Snack: Beet and Walnut Salad

Dinner: Lemon Dill Baked Salmon

Day 23:

Breakfast: Avocado Toast with Poached Egg

Snack: Arugula and Pear Salad

Lunch: Cilantro Lime Chicken Bowl

Snack: Tomato Basil Mozzarella Salad

Dinner: Miso Glazed Salmon

Day 24:

Breakfast: Orange and Ginger Chia Pudding

Snack: Broccoli and Cranberry Salad

Lunch: Kale and Walnut Pesto Pasta

Snack: Chamomile Lavender Tea

Dinner: Garlic Lemon Herb Roasted Vegetables

CONCLUSION

Finally, going on an anti-inflammatory lifestyle path via the perspective of a beginner-friendly cuisine carries the possibility of transforming well-being. The combination of easy-to-follow recipes, nutrition education, and culinary adventure not only simplifies the process but also encourages people to take care of their health.

This cookbook opens the door to a world of brilliant flavors and healthy ingredients, delivering a tasty alternative to inflammation. It demystifies the concept of anti-inflammatory diet for beginners by fusing nutrition science and culinary artistry, making it a manageable and fun endeavor.

One of the most important messages from this cookbook is that following an anti-inflammatory diet does not have to be difficult. Instead, it becomes a gourmet adventure, enabling people to discover the wide range of foods that help to reduce inflammation. Each recipe is a celebration of nutrition that doubles as a gourmet feast, from the rich palette of bright veggies to the healthful goodness of lean meats and heart-healthy fats.

Furthermore, the inclusion of educational components throughout the cookbook elevates it above and beyond a collection of recipes. It is a comprehensive handbook that teaches about the science of inflammation and the enormous impact that dietary choices may have on overall health. This deep understanding enables beginners to make informed food choices, creating a ripple effect that goes beyond the kitchen and into their daily life.

The emphasis on simplicity and accessibility throughout the cookbook, ensuring that even individuals with less cooking experience may embark on this path with confidence. The recipes are developed with novices' busy lifestyles in mind, with quick, easy-to-follow instructions that don't sacrifice flavor or nutritional content. This strategy not only makes it easier to stick to an anti-inflammatory diet, but it also encourages a long-term commitment to improved eating habits.

As they flip through the pages of this cookbook, readers are not only learning to cook, but also establishing a lifestyle that nurtures their bodies from within. The use of anti-inflammatory substances is more than just a fad; it represents a fundamental movement toward holistic well-being. Individuals engage in their health by consuming nutrient-dense, inflammation-fighting foods, laying the groundwork for resilience against chronic illnesses.

This anti-inflammatory cookbook for beginners emerges as a useful thread in the broad tapestry of health and wellness, weaving together dietary concepts, the delights of cooking, and the empowerment of educated choices. It's a road map to robust health, with each recipe serving as a checkpoint and every meal an opportunity to nourish the body and reduce inflammation.

In essence, this cookbook extends an invitation to engage on a revolutionary culinary adventure—one that goes beyond the constraints of traditional diets and welcomes people into a world where health is a continual, savory journey rather than a destination. Beginners who embrace the recipes and thoughts in these pages are building a lifestyle that vibrates with vitality, balance, and a profound sense of well-being, not merely the art of anti-inflammatory cooking.